50 Wart and Fungus Removing and Preventing Meal Recipes:

Quickly and Painlessly Remove Warts and Fungus through All Natural Foods

By

Joe Correa CSN

COPYRIGHT

ACKNOWLEDGEMENTS

This book is dedicated to my friends and family that have had mild or serious illnesses so that you may find a solution and make the necessary changes in your life.

50 Wart and Fungus Removing and Preventing Meal Recipes:

Quickly and Painlessly Remove Warts and Fungus through All Natural Foods

By

Joe Correa CSN

CONTENTS

ABOUT THE AUTHOR

After years of Research, I honestly believe in the positive effects that proper nutrition can have over the body and mind. My knowledge and experience has helped me live healthier throughout the years and which I have shared with family and friends. The more you know about eating and drinking healthier, the sooner you will want to change your life and eating habits.

Nutrition is a key part in the process of being healthy and living longer so get started today. The first step is the most important and the most significant.

INTRODUCTION

50 Wart and Fungus Removing and Preventing Meal Recipes: Quickly and Painlessly Remove Warts and Fungus through All Natural Foods

By Joe Correa CSN

Most people, at least once in their lifetime, suffer from this irritating and sometimes even painful condition often caused by the human papilloma virus (HPV). The manifestation and appearance of warts and fungus depend mostly on the cause and the affected area. Warts and fungus can appear almost anywhere on the body, but most often they choose moist places like small cuts or abrasions on the fingers, hands, and feet. In most cases they are painless, but sometimes they do cause some serious itching and skin irritation.

The biggest question regarding warts and fungus is what's causing warts and fungus to develop. The answer can be quite tricky because of so many factors that directly contribute to this mostly viral infection. Both warts and fungus are extremely contagious and can easily be transmitted from one person to another, or even from one part of the skin to another, especially in small cuts, scratches, or other damaged parts of the skin. They also don't seem to choose any specific age group, but in most cases, kids are especially vulnerable and exposed to their development.

There are, however, a couple of things you can do to prevent this viral infection. The most important thing is to maintain proper hand care and hygiene. This rule goes especially for scratches and open wounds that are prone to infections.

Another important factor is definitely your diet. A healthy diet will build up your immune system and make it strong enough to fight off these infections, which is crucial for warts and fungus removal. Foods rich in vitamin C are proven to help and prevent this condition. Citrus fruits, bell peppers, and berries should be consumed on a daily basis. Another important mineral you simply have to take is Zinc. It can be found in foods like seeds (especially pumpkin seeds), grass-fed beef, and chickpeas. Probiotic rich foods are loaded with good bacteria and will help you restore your natural balance. These foods include dairy products like yogurt, cheese, and fermented vegetables. Leafy greens, loaded with vitamin A, are always a good choice for building up the immune system. As a snack, choose foods high in selenium. This amazing antioxidant is vital for the immune system and can be found in different nuts, especially Brazil nuts. A handful of these nuts will serve as a perfect, healthy snack and will protect you against this irritating problem.

Having this in mind, I have created this meal recipe collection that is based on these healthy foods and will help you boost up your immune system, and prevent these infections once and for all.

50 WART AND FUNGUS REMOVING AND PREVENTING MEAL RECIPES: QUICKLY AND PAINLESSLY REMOVE WARTS AND FUNGUS THROUGH ALL NATURAL FOODS

1.   Carrot Omelet

Ingredients:

5 large eggs, beaten

1 large carrot, sliced

1 tbsp of fresh parsley, finely chopped

2 tbsp of shallots, finely chopped

1 small onion, finely chopped

2 tsp of butter

1 tbsp of skim milk

1 tsp of Himalayan salt

¼ tsp of black pepper, ground

Preparation:

Combine eggs, milk, salt, and pepper in a mixin bowl. Mix well to combine and set aside.

Melt the butter in a large frying pan over a medium-high temperature. Add carrot and cook for 3 minutes. Throw in the shallots and cook for another minute, stirring constantly.

Pour the egg mixture and sprinkle with parsley. Cook for 3 minutes, then flip the omelet. Cook for 2 minutes and remove from the heat. Fold the omelet and serve immediately.

Nutritional information per serving: Kcal: 253, Protein: 17.1g, Carbs: 10.1g, Fats: 16.3g

2.   Tomato-Bean Curry

Ingredients:

2 cups of canned tomatoes, non-salted

1 cup of kidney beans, pre-cooked

1 medium-sized onion, chopped

1 tbsp of olive oil

1 tsp of cumin, ground

½ tsp of ginger, ground

1 garlic clove, minced

1 tsp of curry, ground

1 tsp of salt

Preparation:

Soak the beans overnight or at least for 3 hours. Place them in a pot of boiling water and cook until soften. Remove from the heat and drain well. Set aside.

Preheat the oil in a heavy-bottomed pot over a medium-high temperature. Add garlic, onion, and ginger. Cook for 3-4 minutes, or until translucent.

Now, stir in the tomatoes and beans. Sprinkle with curry and bring it to a boil. Reduce the heat to low and cover with a lid. Cook for 20 minutes or until thick.

Remove from the heat and set aside to cool for a while.

Nutritional information per serving: Kcal: 253, Protein: 17.1g, Carbs: 10.1g, Fats: 16.3g

3.   Oven-Baked Beef Steak

Ingredients:

1 lb of grass-fed beef steak, cut into bite-sized pieces

¼ cup of all-purpose flour

2 cup of canned tomatoes, unsalted

¼ cup of fresh celery, finely chopped

1 large carrot, finely chopped

1 tbsp of Worcestershire sauce

2 tbsp of olive oil

½ tsp of salt

Preparation:

Preheat the oven to 375°F.

Spread the flour over a clean kitchen desk. Place the meat chops and dredge them in flour.

Preheat the oil in a large nonstick skillet over a medium-high temperature. Add meat and cook until golden browned. Remove from the heat and transfer on a large baking sheet. Reserve the pan.

Add celery, carrot, tomatoes, sauce, and salt to the skillet and cook for 5 minutes, stirring constantly. Remove from the heat and pour this mixture over the meat.

Place it in the oven and bake for 1 hour, or until nicely tender.

Nutritional information per serving: Kcal: 253, Protein: 17.1g, Carbs: 10.1g, Fats: 16.3g

4.   Potato Frittata

Ingredients:

1 cup of potatoes, peeled and cubed

2 large red bell peppers, chopped

1 large onion, finely chopped

1 tbsp of vegetable oil

3 large eggs, beaten

½ tsp of salt

Preparation:

Place the potatoes in a pot of boiling water. Cook for 10 minutes, or until tender. Remove from the heat and drain well. Set aside.

Preheat the oil in a large nonstick skillet over a medium-high temperature. Add onions and peppers, and cook for 4-5 minutes, or until fork-tender.

Now, add potatoes and continue to cook until soften and browned. Pour over the eggs and sprinkle with some salt to taste. Cook for another 4-5 minutes and remove from the heat.

Serve warm.

Nutritional information per serving: Kcal: 191, Protein: 8.5g, Carbs: 18.9g, Fats: 9.8g

5.   Hot Tuna Steaks

Ingredients:

1 lb of tuna steaks, boneless

3 tbsp of extra-virgin olive oil

¼ cup of balsamic vinegar

1 tbsp of Dijon mustard

1 tbsp of honey, raw

1 tbsp of fresh rosemary, finely chopped

1 tsp of sea salt

Preparation:

Combine oil, vinegar, honey, mustard, rosemary, and salt in a mixing bowl. Stir well and then add tuna steaks. Coat well with marinade and set aside for 30 minutes to allow flavors to penetrate into the fish.

Now, preheat the grill to a medium-high temperature. Drain the steaks and grill for about 2-3 minutes, or until set.

Pour the remaining marinade into a saucepan and bring it to a boil. Remove from the heat and pour over the steaks. Sprinkle with fresh rosemary.

Serve with some steamed vegetables, but this is optional.

Nutritional information per serving: Kcal: 431, Protein: 45.5g, Carbs: 6.9g, Fats: 23.9g

6.　　Blueberry Breakfast Oatmeal

Ingredients:

1 cup of rolled oats

1 cup of skim milk

½ cup of fresh blueberries

1 tbsp of almonds, roughly chopped

1 tbsp of honey

1 tbsp of sunflower seeds

Preparation:

Combine oatmeals and milk in a large bowl. Heat trough in a microwave and stir in the honey and almonds. Top with blueberries and sunflower seeds.

Serve immediately.

Nutritional information per serving: Kcal: 278, Protein: 10.6g, Carbs: 48.5g, Fats: 5g

7.   Warm Broccoli & Mushroom Salad

Ingredients:

1 lb of fresh broccoli, trimmed

4 oz of button mushrooms, chopped

½ cup of green olives, pitted and chopped

8 oz of cherry tomatoes, chopped

For the dressing:

5 tbsp of extra-virgin olive oil

1 tbsp of red vine vinegar

2 tbsp of lemon juice, freshly squeezed

1 garlic clove, minced

½ tsp of sea salt

½ tsp of black pepper, ground

Preparation:

Combine all dressing ingredients and set aside to allow flavors to mingle.

Place the broccoli in a pot of boiling water and cook for 2 minutes, until fork-tender. Remove from the heat and drain well. Set aside.

Steam the mushrooms for 3-4 minutes, or until tender.

Now, combine broccoli, mushrooms, tomatoes, and olives in a large salad bowl. Pour over the dressing and stir all well to coat. Refrigerate for 20 minutes before serving.

Enjoy!

Nutritional information per serving: Kcal: 176, Protein: 19.3g, Carbs: 47.9g, Fats: 76g

8.   Italian Pasta

Ingredients:

1 lb of whole wheat pasta, pre-cooked

1 large onion, diced

1 cup of tomatoes, diced

1 cup of tomato paste

2 tbsp of fresh parsley, finely chopped

2 garlic clove, minced

1 tsp of fresh basil, finely chopped

1 bay leaf

¼ tsp of black pepper, ground

½ tsp of sea salt

½ tsp of dried oregano, ground

Preparation:

Cook the pasta using package instructions. Remove from the heat and drain well. Set aside.

Preheat a large nonstick saucepan over a medium-high temperature. Pour in the tomatoes, and add garlic, onions, bay leaf, basil, tomato paste, salt, and pepper. Bring it to a boil, then reduce the heat to low and cover with a lid.

Cook for 1 hour, stirring occasionally. Remove from the heat and stir in into the pasta. Sprinkle with some oregano and serve warm.

Nutritional information per serving: Kcal: 399, Protein: 14.2g, Carbs: 81.6g, Fats: 2.7g

9.   Potato Salmon Casserole

Ingredients:

1 lb of wild salmon fillets

1 lb of potatoes, peeled and sliced

4 tbsp of olive oil

½ cup of chicken broth

2 tbsp of balsamic vinegar

1 tbsp of fresh dill, finely chopped

½ cup of sour cream

1 tbsp of horseradish, grated

½ tsp of salt

¼ tsp of black pepper, ground

Preparation:

Preheat the oven to 375°F.

Place the potatoes in a pot of boiling water and cook until fork-tender. Remove from the heat and drain well. Set aside.

Take a large baking sheet and spread the potatoes in one big layer. Top with fillets and sprinkle with olive oil and dill. Cover with aluminum foil and place it in the oven. Bake for 20 minutes. Remove from the oven and drizzle with balsamic vinegar and return to oven for the next 5 minutes, or desired doneness.

Mix together sour cream, horseradish, salt, and pepper. Stir well and pour over the casserole. Set aside for 10 minutes to cool and serve.

Nutritional information per serving: Kcal: 280, Protein: 17.1g, Carbs: 13.5g, Fats: 18.2g

10.   Creamy Spinach Pie

Ingredients:

10 oz of fresh spinach, chopped

1o oz of Cheddar cheese, cubed

2 cups of cottage cheese, crumbled

4 tbsp of butter, melted

5 tbsp of all-purpose flour

6 large eggs, beaten

1 tsp of salt

Preparation:

Preheat the oven to 375°F.

Place the spinach in a pot of boiling water and cook until tender. Remove from the heat and drain well.

Now, combine spinach, cheddar cheese, cottage cheese, butter, flour, and eggs in a large bowl. Sprinkle with some salt and stir all well to blend.

Transfer to a large baking sheet and place it in the oven. Bake for 1 hour, or until crispy edges. Remove from the oven and cut into portions.

Serve immediately.

Nutritional information per serving: Kcal: 432, Protein: 30.5g, Carbs: 10.4g, Fats: 30g

11.   Orange Carrot Smoothie

Ingredients:

1 large carrot, chopped

2 large oranges, peeled

1 egg yolk

1 cup of Greek yoghurt

½ tsp of ginger, ground

1 tbsp of almonds, roughly chopped

Preparation:

Combine all ingredients in a food processor and blend until smooth. Transfer to serving glasses and refrigerate for 1 hour before serving. Garnish with some lemon zest if you like. This is, however, optional.

Enjoy!

Nutritional information per serving: Kcal: 169, Protein: 12.1g, Carbs: 21.4g, Fats: 4.5g

12. Artichoke Rigatoni Pasta

Ingredients:

1 lb of rigatoni pasta

1 cup of artichoke hearts, chopped

3 cups of canned tomatoes, unsalted

4 tbsp of olive oil

1 garlic clove, crushed

1 tbsp of fresh parsley, finely chopped

5 tbsp of Parmesan cheese, grated

¼ tsp of black pepper, ground

½ tsp of salt

Preparation:

Preheat the oil in a large saucepan over a medium-high temperature. Add artichokes and pour over the tomatoes. Sprinkle with parsley and stir well. Cook for 15-20 minutes, stirring occasionally.

Meanwhile, cook the pasta using package instructions. Remove from the heat and drain well. Transfer to a serving dish and pour over the artichoke sauce. Stir all well to coat and sprinkle with cheese, salt, and pepper to taste.

Enjoy!

Nutritional information per serving: Kcal: 399, Protein: 14.2g, Carbs: 81.6g, Fats: 2.7g

13.   Steamed Broccoli with Tomatoes

Ingredients:

10 oz of fresh broccoli, trimmed

2 cups of cherry tomatoes, halved

1 cup of sour cream

4 tbsp of skim milk

½ tsp of curry powder

2 cups of Romaine lettuce, roughly chopped

½ tsp of salt

¼ tsp of black pepper, ground

Preparation:

Steam the broccoli for about 5-7 minutes, or until crisp and tender. Set aside

Meanwhile, combine milk, sour cream, curry, salt, and pepper in a mixing bowl. Pour over the broccoli and place it in the refrigerator for at least 2 hours.

On a serving plate, make a lettuce layer and spoon the broccoli mixture on top. Add tomatoes and sprinkle all with some salt and pepper if needed.

Enjoy!

Nutritional information per serving: Kcal: 139, Protein: 4.2g, Carbs: 10g, Fats: 10g

14.   Smoky Chicken with Carrots & Potato

Ingredients:

2 lbs of chicken breasts, skinless and boneless

2 large carrots, sliced

1 large potato, peeled and cubed

1 tbsp of smoked paprika

1 tsp of onion powder

1 tsp of dried thyme

½ tsp of Cayenne pepper, ground

½ tsp of vegetable seasoning mix

1 tbsp of fresh parsley, finely chopped

½ tsp of black pepper, ground

5 tbsp of olive oil

Preparation:

Preheat the oven to 450°F.

Mix together smoked paprika, onion powder, dried thyme, cayenne pepper, vegetable seasoning mix, black pepper and 2 tablespoons of olive oil in a mixing bowl. Stir well and place the fillets into this mixture. Coat with a spoon from time to time. Let it stand at least for 30 minutes.

Meanwhile, place the potatoes and carrots in a pot of boiling water. Sprinkle with some salt and cook until tender. Remove from the heat and drain.

Transfer to a large baking dish and top with meat. Pour over the marinade and add water enough to cover the bottom of the dish. Place it in the oven and bake for 20-25 minutes, or until golden brown.

Remove from the oven and serve.

Nutritional information per serving: Kcal: 386, Protein: 39g, Carbs: 12.3g, Fats: 19.8g

15. Veal with Avocado-Stuffed Tomatoes

Ingredients:

1 lb of lean veal steaks, boneless

2 tbsp of olive oil

1 tsp of Cayenne pepper, ground

4 large tomatoes, cored

1 cup of avocado, peeled, pitted and chopped

1 medium-sized green bell pepper, chopped

1 tsp of fresh parsley, finely chopped

¼ tsp of chili pepper, ground

¼ tsp of coriander, finely chopped

½ tsp of salt

¼ tsp of black pepper

Preparation:

Preheat the oil in a large frying pan over a medium-high temperature. Add meat and sprinkle with cayenne pepper and salt. Cook for 4-5 minutes, or until desired doneness. Remove from the heat and set aside.

Combine avocado, parsley, chili, coriander, salt, and pepper in a food processor. Blend until nice and creamy. Set aside.

Scoop the tomatoes and spoon the avocado mixture into it. Serve as a side dish with meat.

Nutritional information per serving: Kcal: 249, Protein: 20.2g, Carbs: 8.6g, Fats: 15.4g

16.   Oven-Baked Veggies

Ingredients:

2 small zucchinis, peeled and chopped

1 cup of button mushrooms, chopped

½ cup of cherry tomatoes, halved

1 large bell pepper, chopped

1 medium-sized red onion, sliced

4 tbsp of olive oil

½ tsp of dried basil, ground

½ tsp of salt

¼ tsp of black pepper, ground

2 garlic cloves, crushed

½ tsp of dried oregano, ground

Preparation:

Preheat the oven 400°F.

Combine oil, salt, oregano, garlic, basil, and pepper to a mixing bowl. Mix well and pour this mixture in a large baking dish.

Now, add all prepared vegetables and stir to coat with marinade. Place it in the oven and bake for 20 minutes, or until nicely crisp.

Remove from the oven and serve. Enjoy!

Nutritional information per serving: Kcal: 167, Protein: 2.7g, Carbs: 10.3g, Fats: 14.4g

17.   Chicken Pate with Pecans

Ingredients:

1 lb of chicken fillets, cut into bite-sized pieces

8 oz of cream cheese

1 cup pecans, finely chopped

4 tbsp of mayonnaise

3 tbsp of fresh dill, finely chopped

2 garlic cloves, minced

½ tsp of salt

¼ tsp of Cayenne pepper, ground

1 tbsp of olive oil

Preparation:

Preheat the oil in a large frying pan over a medium-high temperature. Add meat and cook for 5-7 minutes, or until golden brown. Remove from the heat and set aside to cool for a while.

Now, combine chicken with all other ingredients in a food processor. Blend until creamy. Transfer to a serving dish and serve with bread or crackers.

Enjoy!

Nutritional information per serving: Kcal: 385, Protein: 20.9g, Carbs: 6.1g, Fats: 31.7g

18.   Yellow Squash Creamy Bake

Ingredients:

1 medium-sized yellow squash, peeled and seeded

1 cup of Cheddar cheese, grated

1 cup of sour cream

5 tbsp of breadcrumbs

2 large eggs, beaten

2 tbsp of all-purpose flour

½ tsp of salt

¼ tsp of black pepper, ground

Preparation:

Preheat the oven 375°F.

Place the squash chops in a pot of boiling water and cook until fork-tender. remove from the heat and drain. Set aside.

Whisk the eggs, sour cream, flour, salt, and pepper in a mixing bowl.

Grease a large baking sheet with some vegetable oil or a cooking spray. Add squash chops and pour over the sour cream mixture. Sprinkle with cheese and breadcrumbs and place it in the oven. Bake for 20 minutes, or until done.

Nutritional information per serving: Kcal: 419, Protein: 18.3g, Carbs: 14.4g, Fats: 32.6g

19.   Shrimp Paella

Ingredients:

2 lbs of shrimps, cleaned and deveined

1 cup of artichokes, chopped

1 large red bell pepper, chopped

1 medium-sized onion, chopped

1 cup of brown rice

1 cup of frozen peas, thawed

2 garlic cloves, minced

½ tsp of turmeric, ground

½ tsp of smoked paprika, ground

¼ tsp of salt

¼ tsp of black pepper, ground

Preparation:

Place the rice in a deep pot. Add about 3 cups of water and bring it to a boil. Reduce the heat to low and cook for 15 minutes. Remove from the heat and drain. Set aside.

Grease a large skillet with some oil and preheat it to a medium-high temperature. Add onion, garlic, and pepper. Cook for 3-4 minutes, or until pepper soften. Now, add about 3 cups of water and sprinkle with smoked paprika and turmeric. Bring it to a boil then reduce the heat to low. Cover with a lid and cook for 15-20 minutes.

Add shrimps, peas, and artichokes. Cook for 10 more minutes, then stir in the rice. Cook for another 5 minutes, then remove from the heat. Add more salt if needed and serve.

Nutritional information per serving: Kcal: 258, Protein: 29.7g, Carbs: 27.6g, Fats: 2.7g

20.   Potato Carrot Patties

Ingredients:

1 cup of potatoes, peeled and chopped

1 cup of carrots, diced

2 large eggs, beaten

1 cup of breadcrumbs

1 small onion, diced

3 tbsp of all-purpose flour

2 tbsp of olive oil

½ tsp of salt

¼ tsp of Cayenne pepper, ground

Preparation:

Place the potatoes and carrots in a pot of boiling water and cook for 5 minutes. remove from the heat and drain well.

Now, combine potatoes, carrots, eggs, onion, and breadcrumbs in a mixing bowl. Sprinkle with some salt and cayenne pepper and stir well to blend. Form the patties and roll them in flour.

Preheat the oil in a frying pan over a medium-high temperature. Fry the patties for 3-4 minutes on each side, or until golden brown.

Serve with cream cheese or meat. However, this is optional.

Nutritional information per serving: Kcal: 358, Protein: 11.2g, Carbs: 45.9g, Fats: 14.7g

21.   Rotisserie Chicken

Ingredients:

1 lb of chicken breasts, skinless and boneless

2 tbsp of olive oil

4 tbsp of honey, raw

1 tsp of smoked paprika, ground

3 garlic cloves, minced

1 medium-sized onion, diced

1 tsp of salt

¼ tsp of black pepper, ground

½ tsp of dried thyme, ground

Preparation:

Preheat the oven to 350°F.

Combine oil, paprika, honey, onion, garlic, thyme, salt, and pepper in a mixing bowl. Stir well to blend. Rub this marinade into the meat gently into the meat.

Preheat the grill to medium-high temperature. Grill the meat for 45 minutes, or until desired doneness. Using a kitchen brush, soak the meat while grilling.

Remove from the heat and serve immediately.

Nutritional information per serving: Kcal: 474, Protein: 44.6g, Carbs: 28.1g, Fats: 20.7g

22.   Swordfish with Veggies

Ingredients:

1 lb of swordfish steaks, boneless

2 medium-sized tomatoes, sliced

4 oz of button mushrooms, sliced

1 small bell pepper, sliced

1 small onion, chopped

2 tbsp of olive oil

2 tbsp of lemon juice, freshly squeezed

¼ tsp of dried dill, finely chopped

½ tsp of salt

1 bay leaf

Preparation:

Preheat the oven to 400°F.

Combine oil, mushrooms, bell pepper, onion, dill, and lemon juice in a mixing bowl. Stir well to mix and set aside.

On a large baking sheet, spread some aluminum foil. Place the vegetables and top with fish fillets. Cover the fillets with tomatoes and add the bay leaf. Now, take another piece of aluminum foil and wrap all. Place it in the oven and bake for about 50 minutes to 1 hour. The fish is done when it flakes easily with a fork.

Nutritional information per serving: Kcal: 217, Protein: 24.6g, Carbs: 5.9g, Fats: 10.5g

23.   Greens & Citrus Smoothie

Ingredients:

½ cup of fresh spinach, roughly chopped

½ cup of fresh kale, chopped

1 cup of beets, trimmed

2 tbsp of lemon juice, freshly squeezed

2 tbsp of orange juice, freshly squeezed

½ cup of skim milk

2 tbsp of liquid honey

Preparation:

Combine spinach, kale, beets, milk, and honey in a food processor or a blender. Process until smooth and creamy. Transfer to serving glasses and stir in the lemon juice and orange juice.

Add a few ice cubes and serve immediately.

Nutritional information per serving: Kcal: 144, Protein: 4.4g, Carbs: 32.7g, Fats: 0.3g

24.   Corn Avocado Salad

Ingredients:

2 cups of corn, pre-cooked

2 medium-sized bell pepper, ground

1 ripe avocado, pitted, peeled, and chopped

1 medium-sized apple, chopped

3 tbsp of olive oil

1 tbsp of red wine vinegar

2 tsp of Dijon mustard

½ tsp of salt

Preparation:

Place the corn in a pot of boiling water and cook for 10 minutes, or until soften. Remove from the heat and drain. Set aside.

Combine oil, vinegar, mustard, and salt in a mixing bowl. Stir well and set aside.

Now, combine corn, pepper, apple, and avocado in a large salad bowl. Pour over the previously prepared dressing and toss well to coat.

Serve immediately.

Nutritional information per serving: Kcal: 309, Protein: 4.3g, Carbs: 31.2g, Fats: 21.6g

25.   Portobello Provolone

Ingredients:

4 portobello mushrooms, stems removed

4 oz of Provolone cheese, sliced

4 tbsp of balsamic vinegar

1 tbsp of extra-virgin olive oil

2 garlic cloves, minced

1 tsp of dried oregano, ground

1 tsp of dried basil, ground

Preparation:

Combine oil, vinegar, garlic, basil, and oregano in a large bowl. Throw in the mushrooms and coat with this marinade. Let it stand for about 15-20 minutes.

Meanwhile, preheat the grill to medium-high temperature. Grease the grill using a kitchen brush with the marinade.

Grill the mushrooms for about 5-8 minutes, or until golden brown. Sprinkle with cheese in the last minute. Wait until cheese melts, and remove from the grill.

Serve immediately.

Nutritional information per serving: Kcal: 292, Protein: 17.7g, Carbs: 6g, Fats: 22.4g

26.   Tuna Cannellini

Ingredients:

2 cups of cannellini beans, pre-cooked

10 oz of tuna, minced

1 cup of tomatoes, diced

1 small red onion, chopped

2 tbsp of Dijon mustard

2 tbsp of lemon juice, freshly squeezed

4 tbsp of olive oil

½ tsp of sea salt

¼ tsp of black pepper, ground

A handful of fresh basil

Preparation:

Soak the beans overnight.

Drain well and place them in a deep pot. Add 4 cups of water and cook until tender. Remove from the heat and drain. Set aside.

Combine lemon juice, mustard, salt, and pepper in a small bowl.Stir well and gradually add oil. Set aside to meld.

Now, combine previously cooked beans, tuna, onion, and tomatoes in a medium bowl. Drizzle with lemon juice mixture and toss well to coat.

Serve with fresh basil.

Nutritional information per serving: Kcal: 465, Protein: 33.2g, Carbs: 47.4g, Fats: 16.8g

27.   Pumpkin Carrot Soup

Ingredients:

2 cups of yellow pumpkin, cubed

1 medium-sized carrot, chopped

2 cups of chicken broth

1 small onion, chopped

1 garlic clove, minced

¼ tsp of Cayenne pepper, ground

1 tsp of curry powder, ground

1 tsp of olive oil

½ tsp of salt

Preparation:

Preheat the oil in a large saucepan over a medium-high temperature. Add onions and garlic and cook for 3 minutes, or until translucent. Pour in the chicken broth and add pumpkin and carrot. Bring it to a boil and reduce the heat to low. Cover with a lid and cook for 10 minutes more.

Now, transfer to a food processor and blend until creamy. Return to the pot and add cayenne pepper and curry. Stir well and heat it up. Garnish with grated carrot.

Serve immediately.

Nutritional information per serving: Kcal: 70, Protein: 3.4g, Carbs: 11.3g, Fats: 1.8g

28.   Blueberry Beet Smoothie

Ingredients:

1 cup of frozen blueberries

2 medium-sized beets, trimmed

¼ cup of celery, chopped

1 tbsp of honey

1 cup of Greek yogurt

1 tsp of flaxseeds

Preparation:

Combine blueberries, beets, celery, honey, and greek yogurt in a food processor and blend until smooth and creamy. Transfer to serving glasses and sprinkle with flaxseeds.

Enjoy!

Nutritional information per serving: Kcal: 130, Protein: 7.9g, Carbs: 22.4g, Fats: 1.8g

29.   Banana Pancakes

Ingredients:

1 cup of all-purpose flour

1 large banana, chopped

1 tsp of baking powder

½ cup of skim milk

1 large egg

1 tbsp of vegetable oil

¼ tsp of salt

Preparation:

Combine flour, baking powder, and salt in a medium bowl. Stir and set aside.

In a separate bowl, combine milk, banana, and egg. Whisk and pour into a flour mixture. Stir all well until you get a lumpy batter.

Preheat the oil in a frying pan over a medium-high temperature. Spoon about 2 tablespoons of batter to a hot oil and fry for about 2-3 minutes. Flip the pancake and fry for 1 minute more, or until golden brown. Repeat the process with the remaining batter.

Serve pancakes with maple syrup or honey. However, this is optional.

Nutritional information per serving: Kcal: 409, Protein: 12.3g, Carbs: 67.6g, Fats: 10.1g

30.   Navy Turkey Stew

Ingredients:

10 oz of turkey fillets, cut into bite-sized pieces

1 cup of navy beans, soaked overnight

½ cup of white rice

1 small red onion, diced

1 large carrot, diced

1 medium-sized bell pepper, chopped

1 cup of vegetable broth

4 cups of water

¼ tsp of Tabasco sauce

1 celery stalk, chopped

1 tsp of salt

2 tbsp of olive oil

¼ tsp of black pepper, ground

Preparation:

Preheat the oil in a heavy-bottomed pot and add meat chops. Cook for 5 minutes, or until browned, stirring constantly.

Now, add all other ingredients to the pot and bring it to a boil. Reduce the heat to low and cover with a lid. Cook for at least 3 hours.

Serve warm.

Nutritional information per serving: Kcal: 211, Protein: 16g, Carbs: 25g, Fats: 5.3g

31.   Mango Cashew Oatmeal

Ingredients:

1 cup of rolled oats

½ cup of coconut milk

½ cup of mango, chopped

3 tbsp of cashews, roughly chopped

2 tbsp of coconut, shredded

Preparation:

Combine oats and coconut milk in a fire-proof dish. Heat in a microwave and top with mango chops. Sprinkle with coconut and cashews.

Serve immediately.

Nutritional information per serving: Kcal: 435, Protein: 9.6g, Carbs: 48.5g, Fats: 24.9g

32. Perch Spaghetti

Ingredients:

1 lb of perch fillets, boneless

8 oz of spaghetti

2 cups of canned tomatoes, unsalted

2 tbsp of fresh parsley, finely chopped

2 garlic cloves, minced

2 tbsp of lemon juice, freshly squeezed

2 tbsp of apple cider vinegar

2 tbsp of olive oil

½ tsp of Italian seasoning mix

¼ tsp of black pepper, freshly ground

Preparation:

Cut the fillets into bite-sized pieces and set aside.

Cook the spaghetti using package instructions. Remove from the heat and drain well. Set aside.

Preheat the oil in a large skillet over a medium-high temperature. Add garlic, vinegar, and lemon juice. Cook for 2 minutes, stirring constantly.

Now, add chopped fish and cook for 4 minutes, or until almost done. Pour over the tomatoes and sprinkle with parsley, Italian seasoning mix, and pepper. Stir well and bring to a boil. Remove from the heat and pour it all over spaghetti. Toss well to coat and serve immediately.

Nutritional information per serving: Kcal: 303, Protein: 28.5g, Carbs: 28.4g, Fats: 7.9g

33.   Spinach Strawberry Salad

Ingredients:

10 oz of fresh spinach, roughly chopped

10 of fresh strawberries, chopped

1 small onion, sliced

1 small cucumber, sliced

4 tbsp of almonds, roughly chopped

For the dressing:

1 large lemon, juiced

2 tbsp of balsamic vinegar

1 tbsp of olive oil

1 tsp of honey, raw

Preparation:

Combine all dressing ingredients in a mixing bowl and set aside to allow flavors to meld.

Meanwhile, Combine all salad ingredients in a large salad bowl and pour over the dressing. Toss well to coat and refrigerate for 1 hour before serving.

Enjoy!

Nutritional information per serving: Kcal: 115, Protein: 4.2g, Carbs: 12g, Fats: 6.9g

34.   Lentil Carrot Stew

Ingredients:

1 cup of lentils, soaked overnight

3 cups of water

1 tbsp of olive oil

1 garlic clove, crushed

1 small onion, chopped

1 cup of tomatoes, diced

2 medium-sized carrots, sliced

2 medium-sized celery stalks, chopped

½ tsp of salt

¼ tsp of black pepper, ground

Preparation:

Soak the lentils overnight, or at least for 6 hours.

Preheat the oil in a heavy-bottomed pot over a medium-high temperature. Add garlic and onion and stir-fry for 4 minutes, or until translucent.

Add the tomatoes and cook for 1 minute, then add carrots, celery, lentils, and water. Sprinkle with salt and pepper and stir well. You can add chili pepper, if you like it spicier, but this is optional.

Bring it to a boil then reduce the heat to low. Cover with a lid and cook for 1 hour, or until lentils soften.

Nutritional information per serving: Kcal: 153, Protein: 8.9g, Carbs: 23.9g, Fats: 2.7g

35.   Fudgy Cookies

Ingredients:

1 cup of pastry flour

½ cup of cocoa powder, raw

4 large eggs

2 tsp of vanilla extract

½ cup of butter

1tbsp of honey

Preparation:

Preheat the oven to 350°F.

Melt the butter in a microwave or a frying pan. Whisk in the eggs, cocoa, honey, and vanilla extract. Now, add flour and stir all well to combine.

Shape the cookies and place them on a large greased baking sheet.

Place it in the oven and bake for about 20-25 minutes. Remove from the oven and let it cool for a while.

Nutritional information per serving: Kcal: 323, Protein: 9.2g, Carbs: 22.5g, Fats: 23.8g

36.   Morrocan Chicken

Ingredients:

1 lb of chicken breasts, skinless, boneless, and chopped

1 small zucchini, chopped

2 medium-sized bell pepper, chopped

2 cups of tomatoes, diced

10 green olives, pitted and halved

1 tbsp of olive oil

½ tsp of cinnamon, ground

1 tsp of cumin, ground

1 tsp of lemon zest, freshly grated

½ tsp of salt

Preparation:

Preheat the oil in a large skillet over a medium-high temperature. Add meat chops and cook for 5 minutes, or until browned.

Now, add all other ingredients and 1 cup of water. Cook for 20 minutes, or until thickens.

Remove from the heat and serve warm.

Nutritional information per serving: Kcal: 206, Protein: 23.3g, Carbs: 7.3g, Fats: 9.4g

37. Cheese Carrot Balls

Ingredients:

2 cups of carrots, shredded

8 oz of cream cheese

2 cup of Cheddar cheese, shredded

1 tsp of Worcestershire sauce

2 tbsp of fresh parsley, finely chopped

2 oz of pecans, finely chopped

2 oz of almonds, finely chopped

Preparation:

Combine Cheddar cheese, cream cheese, sauce, and carrots in a large bowl. Stir well to combine. Cover with a foil and refrigerate for 1 hour.

Shape the balls and roll them in nuts. Wrap in waxed paper and refrigerate for again for 2 hours before serving.

Enjoy!

Nutritional information per serving: Kcal: 360, Protein: 13.4g, Carbs: 7.5g, Fats: 31.9g

38.   Green Rice

Ingredients:

2 cups of white rice

10 oz of fresh spinach, chopped

5 tbsp of Parmesan cheese, grated

5 tbsp of olive oil

2 garlic cloves, minced

4 tbsp of almonds, chopped

4 tbsp of fresh parsley, finely chopped

½ tsp of salt

¼ tsp of black pepper, ground

Preparation:

Place rice in a deep pot. Add 5 cups of water and bring it to a boil. Reduce the heat to low and cover with a lid. Cook for 15 minutes and remove from the heat. Transfer to a serving bowl and set aside.

Combine spinach, cheese, oil, garlic, almonds, salt, and pepper in a food processor. Blend until smooth and creamy and pour over the rice. Stir well to coat and sprinkle with parsley.

Serve immediately.

Nutritional information per serving: Kcal: 582, Protein: 14.1g, Carbs: 79.1g, Fats: 24.1g

39. Mushroom Crostini

Ingredients:

1 cup of button mushrooms, chopped

1 cup of carrots, sliced

1 tbsp of fresh parsley, finely chopped

1 tbsp of olive oil

2 garlic cloves, minced

1 small onion, chopped

12 slices of bread, toasted

Preparation:

Preheat the oil in a large skillet over a medium-high temperature. Add onion and garlic and stir-fry for 4 minutes, or until translucent. Add mushrooms and cook for 10 minutes. Reduce the heat to low and stir in the parsley. Cook for another minute and remove from the heat. Set aside to cool for a while.

Toast the bread to lightly brown. Place the mushrooms mixture between the two bread slices and serve.

Nutritional information per serving: Kcal: 582, Protein: 14.1g, Carbs: 79.1g, Fats: 24.1g

40.   Stuffed Eggs with Chickpeas

Ingredients:

4 large eggs, hard-boiled

½ cup of chickpeas, pre-cooked

1 tbsp of Greek yogurt

1 tsp of Dijon mustard

1 garlic clove, minced

Preparation:

Place the chickpeas in a pot of boiling water. Cook until tender and remove from the heat and drain well. Set aside.

Gently place the eggs in a pot of boiling water. Add a pinch of salt for easier peeling. Cook for 10 minutes and remove from the heat. Let it cool completely, then peel them.

Cut the eggs in half and discard yolks. Set aside.

Combine chickpeas, yogurt, mustard, and garlic in a food processor. Process until creamy. Spoon this mixture into the egg halves. Serve immediately.

Nutritional information per serving: Kcal: 397, Protein: 31.5g, Carbs: 35.4g, Fats: 14.9g

41.   Okra with Rice

Ingredients:

2 cups of fresh okra, chopped

2 cups of chicken broth

2 cups of canned tomatoes

1 large bell pepper, chopped

1 small onion, chopped

1 cup of white rice

½ tsp of salt

¼ tsp of Cayenne pepper, ground

½ tsp of black pepper, ground

1 tbsp of olive oil

Preparation:

Preheat the oil in a large nonstick skillet over a medium-high temperature. Add okra and cook for 5 minutes, or until lightly browned. Add onion and peppers and cook until vegetables are fork-tender.

Pour in the chicken broth and add rice. Bring it to a boil then reduce the heat to low and cover with a lid. Cook for about 15-20 minutes, or until almost dried out. Now, add tomatoes and sprinkle with cayenne pepper, black pepper, and salt to taste. Cook for 2 minutes, or until heated trough.

Remove from the heat and serve warm.

Nutritional information per serving: Kcal: 155, Protein: 4.6g, Carbs: 27.9g, Fats: 2.8g

42. Cranberry Honey Smoothie

Ingredients:

½ cup of frozen cranberries

1 large egg

1 tsp of vanilla extract

1 cup of Greek yogurt

1 tbsp of honey

A few mint leaves

Preparation:

Combine all ingredients in a food processor or a blender. Blend until nice and creamy. Transfer to serving glasses and add a few ice cubes. Garnish with mint leaves before serving.

Nutritional information per serving: Kcal: 159, Protein: 12.5g, Carbs: 15.3g, Fats: 4.4g

43.   Pepper Potato Frittata

Ingredients:

1 small potato, peeled and thinly sliced

1 small bell pepper, chopped

1 small onion, chopped

5 large eggs

4 tbsp of Gouda cheese, grated

½ tsp of Himalayan salt

¼ tsp of black pepper, ground

Preparation:

Preheat the oven to 375°F.

Preheat the oil in a frying pan over a medium-high temperature. Add potato, bell pepper, and onion and cook for 5 minutes, or until all nicely soften. Remove from the heat and transfer all to a small casserole dish.

Beat the eggs, salt, and pepper in a mixing bowl and pour over the vegetables. Place it in the oven and bake for 20 minutes, or until eggs are set. Remove from the oven and cut into portions.

Enjoy!

Nutritional information per serving: Kcal: 239, Protein: 16g, Carbs: 16.2g, Fats: 12.6g

44.   Couscous with Veggies

Ingredients:

1 cup of couscous

2 cups of chicken broth

1 small onion, chopped

1 medium-sized bell pepper, chopped

1 medium-sized celery stalk, chopped

2 garlic cloves, crushed

1 tbsp of fresh parsley, finely chopped

½ tsp of salt

¼ tsp of chili pepper, ground

1 tbsp of olive oil

Preparation:

Preheat the oil in a large skillet over a medium-high temperature. Add onion, bell pepper, celery, and garlic. Cook for 4 minutes, or until tender.

Pour in the broth and bring it to a boil. Add couscous and stir well. Cook for 1 minute and remove from the heat. Let it stand for 15 minutes until couscous soaks up the liquid. Fluf with a fork and serve.

Nutritional information per serving: Kcal: 232, Protein: 8.6g, Carbs: 38.6g, Fats: 4.6g

45. Slow Cooked Beef Stew

Ingredients:

1 lb of beef steak, cut into bite-sized pieces

2 cups of canned tomatoes

1 tbsp of olive oil

4 oz of button mushrooms, chopped

4 tbsp of tomato paste

1 small onion, chopped

2 garlic cloves, crushed

½ tsp of salt

¼ tsp of black pepper, ground

Preparation:

Grease a slow cooker with the oil. Place the meat chops on the bottom of the cooker. Now, pour the tomatoes, mushrooms, onion, and garlic. Add water enough to cover all ingredients. Seal the lid of the cooker and set to cook for 8-10 hours.

Remove from the heat and open the lid and stir in the tomato paste. Cook for 10 minutes, stirring occasionally.

Serve warm.

Nutritional information per serving: Kcal: 229, Protein: 29.6g, Carbs: 7.8g, Fats: 8.7g

46.   Pasta with Tuna

Ingredients:

1 lb of whole wheat pasta, pre-cooked

1 can of tuna, minced

5 oz of green beans

5 oz of artichokes, chopped

4 tbsp of Parmesan cheese, grated

1 tbsp of lemon juice, freshly juiced

½ tsp of salt

¼ tsp of black pepper, freshly ground

Preparation:

Cook pasta using package instructions. Remove from the heat and drain well.

Place green beans and artichokes in a pot of boiling water. Cook until tender and remove from the heat. Drain well and transfer to a large bowl. Add tuna and sprinkle with salt and pepper. Stir all well to combine. Pour this mixture into the bowl with pasta and toss well to coat. Drizzle with lemon juice and top with parmesan cheese.

Enjoy!

Nutritional information per serving: Kcal: 456, Protein: 25.3g, Carbs: 72.3g, Fats: 7.5g

47.   Stuffed Pita Breads

Ingredients:

1 cup of broccoli, chopped

1 cup of Swiss cheese, shredded

½ cup of cauliflower, chopped

1 medium-sized carrot, sliced

1 small onion, chopped

1 cup of tomatoes, diced

1 tbsp of butter

¼ tsp of dried oregano, ground

4 whole pitas, halved

Preparation:

Melt the butter in a large nonstick skillet over a medium-high temperature. Throw in the broccoli, carrot, cauliflower, and onion. Cook for 4 minutes, or until fork-tender. remove from the heat and transfer to a large bowl. Stir in the tomatoes, cheese, and sprinkle with oregano. Toss well to coat and spoon into pita halves.

Serve immediately.

Nutritional information per serving: Kcal: 326, Protein: 14.4g, Carbs: 42g, Fats: 11.3g

48.   Creamy Omelet

Ingredients:

6 large eggs, beaten

1 large red bell pepper, ground

½ cup of cream cheese

1 tbsp of butter

3 tbsp of shallots, minced

1 tbsp of Parmesan cheese, grated

½ tsp of dried oregano, ground

½ tsp of sea salt

¼ tsp of black pepper, ground

Preparation:

Whisk eggs, cheese, shallots, oregano, salt, and pepper in a mixing bowl.

Melt the butter in a large frying pan over a medium-high temperature. Add peppers and onion and cook for 3-4 minutes, or until crisp-tender. Pour the egg mixture and cook for 5 minutes, or until eggs are set.

Remove from the heat and fold the omelet and serve.

Nutritional information per serving: Kcal: 532, Protein: 27.6g, Carbs:10.5g, Fats: 43.2g

49.   Pineapple Oatmeal

Ingredients:

1 cup of rolled oats

½ cup of pineapple chunks

½ cup of skim milk

½ tsp of cinnamon, ground

A few mint leaves, roughly chopped

Preparation:

Combine oats and milk and heat it up in a microwave. Stir in the cinnamon and top with pineapple. Sprinkle with fresh mint and serve immediately.

Nutritional information per serving: Kcal: 532, Protein: 27.6g, Carbs:10.5g, Fats: 43.2g

50.   Poached Salmon with Carrots

Ingredients:

1 lb of salmon fillets

1 small onion, sliced

1 medium-sized carrot, sliced

2 tbsp of lemon juice, freshly juiced

2 tbsp of olive oil

1 tbsp of fresh dill, finely chopped

4 cups of water

½ tsp of salt

¼ tsp of black pepper, ground

Preparation:

Preheat the oven to 375°F.

Pour the water in a deep pot. Add onion, carrot, lemon juice, oil, dill, salt, and pepper. Bring it to a boil then reduce the heat to low. Cook for 5 minutes more and remove from the heat.

Place the salmon in a large baking dish in one layer. Pour over the previously cooked mixture. Cover with a lid or wrap with aluminum foil.

Place it in the oven and bake for 15-20 minutes. Remove from the heat and serve.

Nutritional information per serving: Kcal: 130, Protein: 12.9g, Carbs: 2.2g, Fats: 8.1g

ADDITIONAL TITLES FROM THIS AUTHOR

70 Effective Meal Recipes to Prevent and Solve Being Overweight: Burn Fat Fast by Using Proper Dieting and Smart Nutrition

By

Joe Correa CSN

48 Acne Solving Meal Recipes: The Fast and Natural Path to Fixing Your Acne Problems in Less Than 10 Days!

By

Joe Correa CSN

41 Alzheimer's Preventing Meal Recipes: Reduce or Eliminate Your Alzheimer's Condition in 30 Days or Less!

By

Joe Correa CSN

70 Effective Breast Cancer Meal Recipes: Prevent and Fight Breast Cancer with Smart Nutrition and Powerful Foods

By

Joe Correa CSN

www.ingramcontent.com/pod-product-compliance
Lightning Source LLC
Chambersburg PA
CBHW051031030426
42336CB00015B/2826